Fit and Healthy Comfort Food Cooking Guide for Beginners

My favourite super simple comfort food recipe collection

Jordan Viking

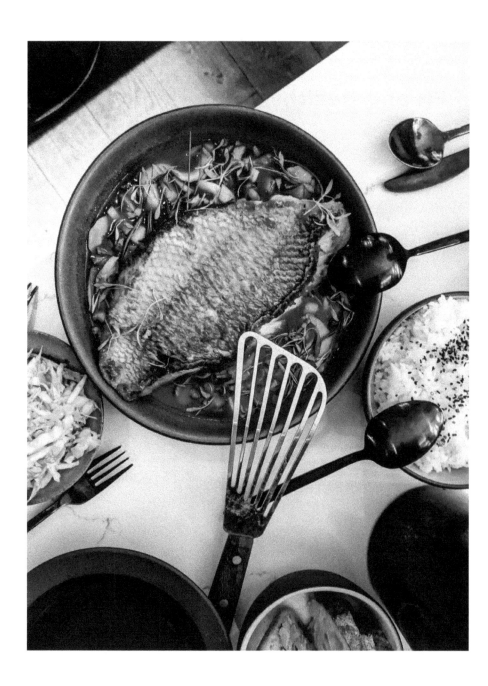

professional advice. The content within this book has been derived from various sources. Please consult a licensed professional before attempting any techniques outlined in this book.

By reading this document, the reader agrees that under no circumstances is the author responsible for any losses, direct or indirect, which are incurred as a result of the use of information contained within this document, including, but not limited to, — errors, omissions, or inaccuracies.

Table of Contents

Parmesan Shrimp Risotto

Preparation Time: 10 minutes | Cooking Time: 6 minutes | Servings: 6

Ingredients:

1 lb jumbo shrimp, deveined and uncooked

1 lb Arborio rice

1 tbsp butter

1 tbsp olive oil

1/2 onion, diced

1 tbsp garlic, minced

1/2 cup peas

1 3/4 cups parmesan cheese, grated

8 cups chicken broth

Directions:

Add butter and oil into the inner pot of Pressure Pot duo crisp and set pot on sauté mode.

Add onion and garlic and cook for 2-3 minutes.

Add shrimp and cook until just opaque. Remove shrimp from pot and set aside.

Add broth and rice. Stir well.

Seal the pot with a pressure-cooking lid and cook on high for 6 minutes.

Once done, allow to release pressure naturally. Remove lid.

Stir in parmesan cheese, peas, and shrimp.

Serve and enjoy.

Nutrition:

Calories 464, Fat 8.3g, Carbohydrates 66.3g, Sugar 3.4g, Protein 28.6g, Cholesterol 166mg.

Asparagus Shrimp Risotto

Preparation time: 10 minutes | Cooking Time: 16 minutes | Servings: 6

Ingredients:

1 1/2 cups arborio rice

1 tbsp butter

3 1/2 cups chicken stock

1/2 cup white wine

1 cup mushrooms, sliced

1/4 cup parmesan cheese, grated

1 lb shrimp, cooked

1 cup asparagus, chopped

1/2 onion, diced

2 tsp olive oil

1/2 tsp pepper

Salt

Directions:

Add oil into the Pressure Pot and set the pot on sauté mode.

Add onion to the pot and sauté for 2-3 minutes.

Add mushrooms and cook for 5 minutes.

Add rice and cook until lightly brown.

Add stock and wine and stir well.

Seal pot with lid and cook on manual high pressure for 6 minutes,

Once done then release pressure using the quick-release method then open the lid.

Add asparagus and butter and cook on sauté mode for 1 minute.

Add shrimp and cook for 1 minute.

Stir in cheese and serve.

Nutrition:

Calories 339, Fat 6.4g, Carbohydrates 42.3g, Sugar 1.6g, Protein 23.3g, Cholesterol 168mg.

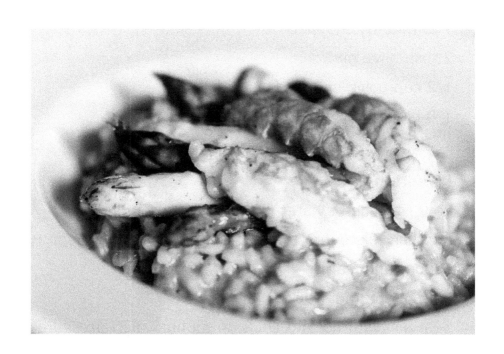

Basil Tilapia

Preparation time: 10 minutes | Cooking Time: 4 minutes | Servings: 4

Ingredients:

4 tilapia fillets

3 garlic cloves, minced

2 tomatoes, chopped

2 tbsp olive oil

1/2 cup basil, chopped

1/8 tsp pepper

1/4 tsp salt

Directions:

Pour half cup of water into the Pressure Pot.

Add fish fillets into the steamer basket and season with pepper and salt.

Place a steamer basket into the pot.

Seal pot with lid and cook on manual high pressure for 2 minutes.

Once done then release pressure using the quick-release method then open the lid.

In a bowl, mix tomatoes, basil, oil, garlic, pepper, and salt.

Place cooked fish fillets on serving plate and top with tomato mixture.

Serve and enjoy.

Nutrition:

Calories 168, Fat 8.2g, Carbohydrates 3.3g, Sugar 1.7g, Protein 21.8g, Cholesterol 55mg.

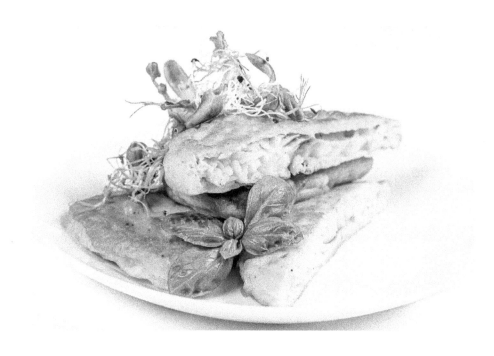

Delicious Shrimp Risotto

Preparation time: 10 minutes | Cooking Time: 17 minutes | Servings: 4

Ingredients:

1 lb. shrimp, peeled, deveined, and chopped

1 1/2 cups arborio rice

1/2 tbsp paprika

1/2 tbsp oregano, minced

1 red pepper, chopped

1 onion, chopped

1/2 cup parmesan cheese, grated

1 cup clam juice

3 cups chicken stock

1/4 cup dry sherry

2 tbsp butter

1/4 tsp pepper

1/2 tsp salt

Directions:

Add butter into the Pressure Pot and set the pot on sauté mode.

Add onion and pepper and sauté until onion is softened.

Add paprika, oregano, pepper, and salt. Stir for a minute.

Add rice and stir for a minute.

Add sherry, clam juice, and stock. Stir well.

Seal pot with lid and cook on manual high pressure for 10 minutes.

Once done then release pressure using the quick-release method then open the lid.

Add shrimp and cook on sauté mode for 2 minutes.

Stir in cheese and serve.

Nutrition:

Calories 530, Fat 10.4g, Carbohydrates 71.6g, Sugar 5.3g, Protein 34.5g, Cholesterol 259mg.

Cajun shrimp

Preparation time: 10 minutes | Cooking Time: 2 minutes | Servings: 4

Ingredients:

1 lb. shrimp, peeled and deveined

15 asparagus spears

1 tbsp cajun seasoning

1 tsp olive oil

Directions:

Pour 1 cup of water into the Pressure Pot then place the steam rack inside the pot.

Arrange asparagus on a steam rack in a layer.

Place shrimp on the top of asparagus.

Sprinkle cajun seasoning over shrimp and drizzle with olive oil.

Seal pot with lid and cook on steam mode for 2 minutes.

Once done then release pressure using the quick-release method then open the lid.

Serve and enjoy.

Nutrition:

Calories 163, Fat 3.2g, Carbohydrates 5.2g, Sugar 1.7g, Protein 27.8g, Cholesterol 239mg.

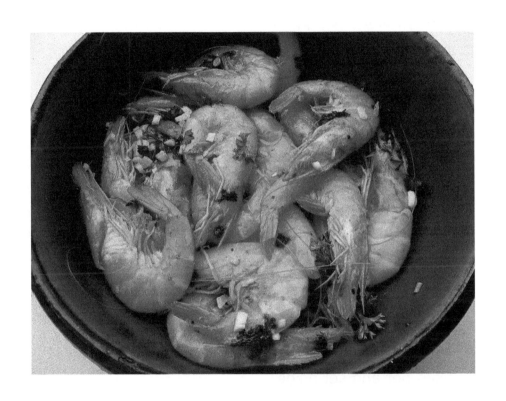

Tomato Beef Brisket

Preparation Time: 10 minutes | Cooking Time: 6 hours 10 minutes | Servings: 6

Ingredients:

3 lbs beef brisket

1 large onion, chopped

1 cup chicken stock

28 oz can tomato, diced

2 tbsp olive oil

4 garlic cloves, minced

Pepper

Salt

Directions:

Season meat with pepper and salt.

Add oil into the inner pot of Pressure Pot duo crisp and set pot on sauté mode.

Add meat to the pot and cook until browned. Remove from pot and set aside.

Add remaining oil to the pot.

Add onion and sauté until softened.

Return meat to the pot.

Top with tomatoes, garlic, pepper, salt, and stock.

Seal the pot with a pressure-cooking lid and select slow cook mode and cook on low for 6 hours.

Slice and serve.

Nutrition:

Calories 504, Fat 18g, Carbohydrates 9g, Sugar 5g, Protein 70g, Cholesterol 203mg.

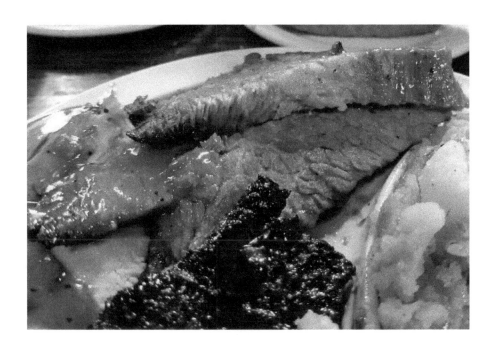

Balsamic Chuck Roast

Preparation Time: 10 minutes | Cooking Time: 55 minutes | Servings: 6

Ingredients:

3 lbs chuck roast

1 tbsp butter, melted

1 tsp rosemary

1 tbsp olive oil

1 cup chicken stock

4 tbsp balsamic vinegar

1/4 tsp thyme, dried

1/2 tsp pepper

1 tsp salt

Directions:

In a small bowl, mix thyme, rosemary, pepper, and salt and rub over meat.

Add oil into the inner pot of Pressure Pot duo crisp and set pot on sauté mode.

Place meat in the pot and cook until brown, about 5 minutes on each side.

Pour broth, butter, and vinegar over meat.

Seal the pot with a pressure-cooking lid and cook on high 40 for minutes.

Once done, release pressure using a quick release. Remove lid.

Serve and enjoy.

Nutrition:

Calories 532, Fat 23g, Carbohydrates 0.5g, Sugar 0.2g, Protein 75g, Cholesterol 234mg.

Classic Pot Roast

Preparation Time: 10 minutes | Cooking Time: 55 minutes | Servings: 6

Ingredients:

3 lbs beef chuck roast

2 tbsp butter

1 tbsp Italian seasoning

2 garlic cloves, minced

4 large carrots, peeled

2 cups chicken stock

1 onion, diced

1 tsp black pepper

1 tsp salt

Directions:

Place meat in a large dish and sprinkle with spices.

Add oil into the inner pot of Pressure Pot duo crisp and set pot on sauté mode.

Add onion and sauté for 5 minutes.

Add meat and stock and stir well.

Seal the pot with a pressure-cooking lid and cook on high for 40 minutes.

Once done, release pressure using a quick release. Remove lid.

Add carrots and stir well.

Seal the pot with a pressure-cooking lid and cook on high for 10 minutes.

Once done, release pressure using a quick release. Remove lid.

Stir and serve.

Nutrition:

Calories 897, Fat 67g, Carbohydrates 7g, Sugar 3g, Protein 60g, Cholesterol 245mg

Quick & easy shrimp

Preparation time: 10 minutes | Cooking Time: 1 minute | Servings: 6

Ingredients:

30 oz frozen shrimp, deveined

1/2 cup chicken stock

1/2 cup apple cider vinegar

Directions:

Add all ingredients into the Pressure Pot and stir well.

Seal pot with lid and cook on manual high pressure for 1 minute.

Once done then release pressure using the quick-release method then open the lid.

Serve and enjoy.

Nutrition:

Calories 156, Fat 2.6g, Carbohydrates 1.5g, Sugar 0.1g, Protein 29g, Cholesterol 213mg.

Cheesy Shrimp Grits

Preparation time: 10 minutes | Cooking Time: 7 minutes | Servings: 6

Ingredients:

1 lb shrimp, thawed

1/2 cup cheddar cheese, shredded

1/2 cup quick grits

1 tbsp butter

1 1/2 cups chicken broth

1/4 tsp red pepper flakes

1/2 tsp paprika

2 tbsp cilantro, chopped

1 tbsp coconut oil

1/2 tsp kosher salt

Directions:

Add oil into the Pressure Pot and set the pot on sauté mode.

Add shrimp and cook until shrimp is no longer pink. Season with red pepper flakes and salt.

Remove shrimp from the pot and set aside.

Add remaining ingredients into the pot and stir well.

Seal pot with lid and cook on manual high pressure for 7 minutes.

Once done then allow to release pressure naturally then open the lid.

Stir in cheese and top with shrimp.

Nutrition:

Calories 221, Fat 9.1g, Carbohydrates 12g, Sugar 0.3g, Protein 21.9g, Cholesterol 174mg.

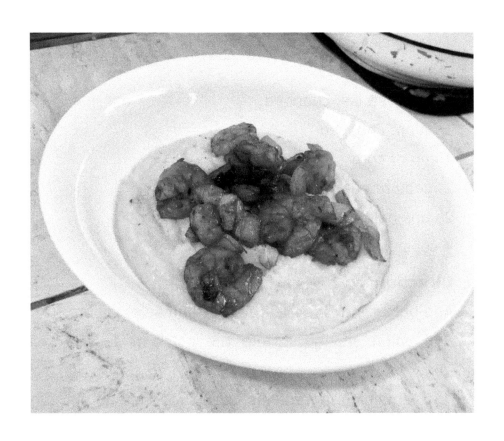

Healthy Salmon Chowder

Preparation time: 10 minutes | Cooking Time: 8 minutes | Servings: 4

Ingredients:

1 lb frozen salmon

2 garlic cloves, minced

2 tbsp butter

2 celery stalks, chopped

1 onion, chopped

1 cup of corn

1 medium potato, cubed

2 cups half and half

4 cups chicken broth

Directions:

Add butter into the Pressure Pot and select sauté.

Add onion and garlic into the pot and sauté for 3-4 minutes.

Add remaining ingredients except for the half and a half and stir well.

Seal pot with lid and cook on manual high pressure for 5 minutes.

Once done then allow to release pressure naturally then open the lid.

Add half and half and stir well.

Serve and enjoy.

Nutrition:

Calories 571, Fat 35.1g, Carbohydrates 26g, Sugar 3.9g, Protein 36.9g, Cholesterol 133mg.

Shrimp with sausage

Preparation time: 10 minutes | Cooking Time: 5 minutes | Servings: 6

Ingredients:

1 lb frozen shrimp

1 1/2 cups sausage, sliced

3 ears corn, cut in thirds

1 lemon, wedges

2 cups chicken broth

1 1/2 tbsp old bay seasoning

1/4 cup parsley, chopped

5 small potatoes, diced

2 garlic cloves, minced

1 onion, chopped

Directions:

Add all ingredients into the Pressure Pot and stir well.

Seal pot with lid and cook on manual high pressure for 5 minutes.

Once done then release pressure using the quick-release method then open the lid.

Serve and enjoy.

Nutrition:

Calories 290, Fat 4.8g, Carbohydrates 40.1g, Sugar 5.2g, Protein 23.6g, Cholesterol 119mg.

Parmesan Salmon

Preparation time: 10 minutes | Cooking Time: 15 minutes | Servings: 4

Ingredients:

4 salmon fillets

1/4 cup parmesan cheese, grated

1/2 cup walnuts

1 tsp olive oil

1 tbsp lemon rind

Directions:

Line Pressure Pot air fryer basket with parchment paper.

Place salmon fillets on parchment paper in an air fryer basket.

Add walnuts into the food processor and process until finely ground.

Mix ground walnuts, cheese, oil, and lemon rind.

Spoon walnut mixture over the salmon fillets and press gently.

Place air fryer basket in the pot.

Seal the pot with an air fryer lid and select bake mode and cook at 400° f for 15 minutes.

Serve and enjoy.

Nutrition:

Calories 349, Fat 21.8g, Carbohydrates 1.9g, Sugar 0.3g, Protein 38.9g, Cholesterol 80mg.

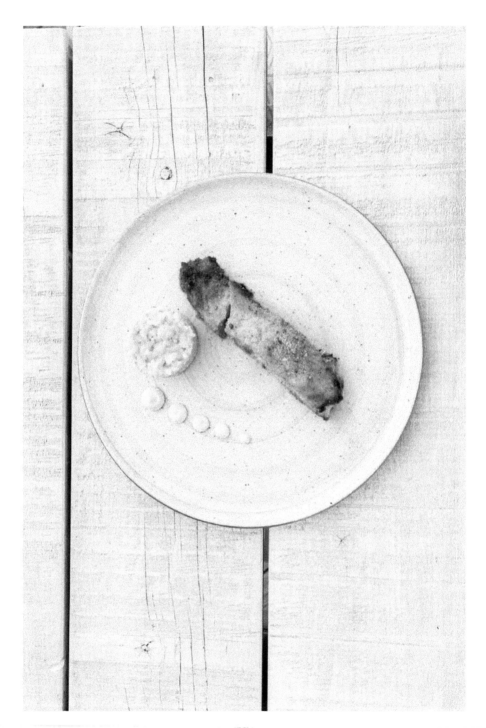

Delicious Pesto Salmon

Preparation time: 10 minutes | Cooking Time: 20 minutes | Servings: 2

Ingredients:

2 salmon fillets

1/4 cup parmesan cheese, grated

For pesto:

1/4 cup olive oil

1 1/2 cups fresh basil leaves

3 garlic cloves, peeled and chopped

1/4 cup parmesan cheese, grated

1/4 cup pine nuts

1/4 tsp black pepper

1/2 tsp salt

Directions:

Add all pesto ingredients into the blender and blend until smooth.

Line Pressure Pot air fryer basket with parchment paper.

Place salmon fillet on parchment paper in the air fryer basket.

Spread 2 tablespoons of the pesto on each salmon fillet.

Sprinkle cheese on top of the pesto.

Place basket in the pot.

Seal the pot with an air fryer lid and select bake mode and cook at 400° f for 20 minutes.

Serve and enjoy.

Nutrition:

Calories 589, Fat 48.7g, Carbohydrates 4.5g, Sugar 0.7g, Protein 38.9g, Cholesterol 81mg.

Crisp & Delicious Catfish

Preparation time: 10 minutes | Cooking Time: 20 minutes | Servings: 2

Ingredients:

2 catfish fillets

1/4 cup cornmeal

1/2 tsp garlic powder

1/2 tsp onion powder

1/2 tsp salt

Directions:

Add cornmeal, garlic powder, onion powder, and salt into a zip-lock bag.

Add fish fillets to the zip-lock bag. Seal bag and shake gently to coat fish fillet.

Line Pressure Pot air fryer basket with parchment paper.

Place coated fish fillets on parchment paper in the air fryer basket. Place basket in the pot.

Seal the pot with an air fryer lid and select air fry mode and cook at 400° f for 20 minutes. Turn fish fillets halfway through.

Serve and enjoy.

Nutrition:

Calories 276, Fat 12.7g, Carbohydrates 12.7g, Sugar 0.5g, Protein 26.3g, Cholesterol 75mg.

Easy Paprika Salmon

Preparation time: 10 minutes | Cooking Time: 7 minutes | Servings: 2

Ingredients:

2 salmon fillets, remove any bones

2 tsp paprika

2 tsp olive oil

Pepper

Salt

Directions:

Brush each salmon fillet with oil, paprika, pepper, and salt.

Line Pressure Pot air fryer basket with parchment paper.

Place salmon fillets on parchment paper in the air fryer basket. Place basket in the pot.

Seal the pot with an air fryer lid and select air fry mode and cook at 390° F for 7 minutes.

Serve and enjoy.

Nutrition:

Calories 282, Fat 15.9g, Carbohydrates 1.2g, Sugar 0.2g, Protein 34.9g, Cholesterol 78mg.

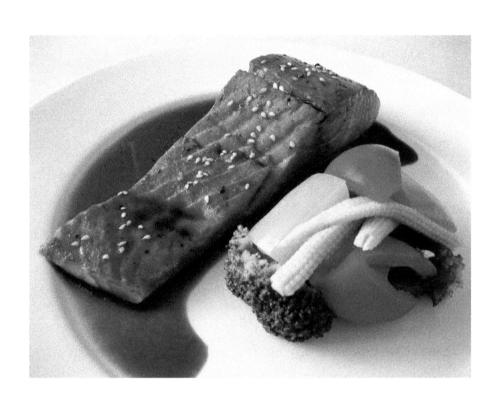

Ranch fish fillets

Preparation time: 10 minutes | Cooking Time: 12 minutes | Servings: 2

Ingredients:

2 fish fillets

1 egg, lightly beaten

1 1/4 tbsp olive oil

1/4 cup breadcrumbs

1/2 packet ranch dressing mix

Directions:

In a shallow dish, mix breadcrumbs, ranch dressing mix, and oil.

Dip fish fillet in egg then coats with breadcrumb mixture and place on parchment paper in the air fryer basket. Place basket in the pot.

Seal the pot with an air fryer lid and select air fry mode and cook at 400° f for 12 minutes.

Serve and enjoy.

Nutrition:

Calories 373, Fat 22.9g, Carbohydrates 25.7g, Sugar 1.2g, Protein 18g, Cholesterol 113mg.

Teriyaki Kababs

Preparation Time: 10 minutes | Cooking Time: 10 minutes | Servings: 4

Ingredients:

1 lb top sirloin steak, boneless and cut into 1-inch cubes

1 onion, diced

1 cup cherry tomatoes

1 bell pepper, cut into 1-inch pieces

1 cup teriyaki sauce

Directions:

Add meat and teriyaki sauce into the mixing bowl. Mix well and place in the refrigerator for 1 hour.

Thread marinated meat, cherry tomatoes, onion, and bell pepper on soaked wooden skewers.

Spray Pressure Pot multi-level air fryer basket with cooking spray.

Place skewers into the air fryer basket and place basket into the Pressure Pot.

Seal pot with air fryer lid and select air fry mode then set the temperature to 400° F and timer for 10 minutes. Turn skewers halfway through.

Serve and enjoy.

Nutrition:

Calories 303, Fat 7.3g, Carbohydrates 17.8g, Sugar 14g, Protein 39.7g, Cholesterol 101mg

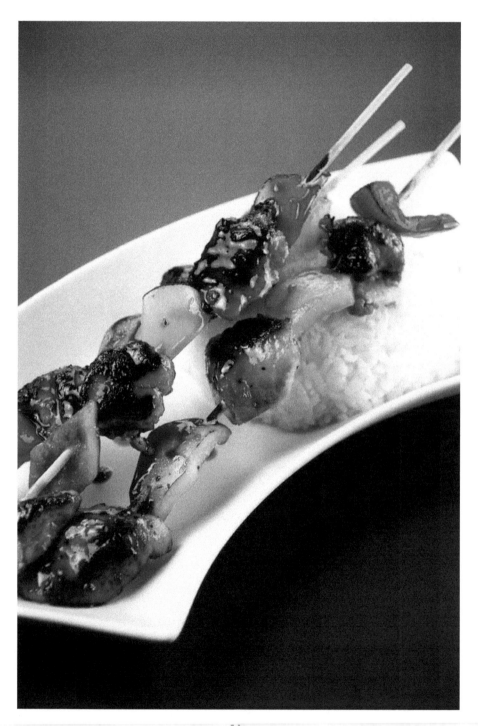

Cheesy Potato Casserole

Preparation Time: 10 minutes | Cooking Time: 45 minutes | Servings: 8

Ingredients:

2 lbs hash browns

3 cups cheddar cheese, shredded

1/2 cup onion, chopped

1/2 cup butter, melted

2 cups sour cream

1 cup cream of chicken soup

Pepper

Salt

2 cups corn flakes, crushed

1/2 cup butter, melted

Directions:

Spray Pressure Pot from inside with cooking spray.

In a large bowl, mix all ingredients except 2 cups cheddar cheese and pour into the Pressure Pot, and spread well.

Sprinkle 2 cups cheddar cheese on top.

Mix crushed corn flakes and butter and sprinkle on top of the cheese.

Seal pot with air fryer lid and select bake mode then set the temperature to 350° F and timer for 45 minutes. Serve and enjoy.

Nutrition:

Calories 854, Fat 65.1g, Carbohydrates 51.8g, Sugar 3g, Protein 17.3g, Cholesterol 133mg.

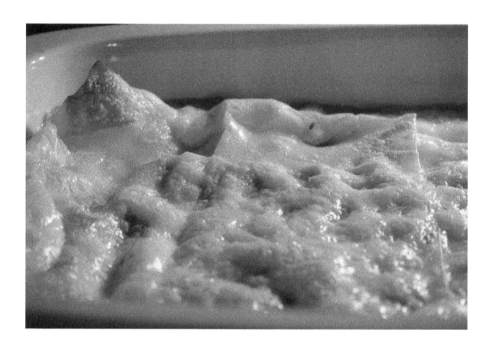

Salmon and Black Olives Mix

Preparation time: 5 minutes | Cooking Time: 15 minutes | Servings: 4

Ingredients:

1 pound salmon fillets, boneless, skinless, and cubed

1 cup black olives, pitted and chopped

1 cup kalamata olives, pitted and chopped

2 garlic cloves, minced

1 tablespoon olive oil

A pinch of salt and black pepper

¼ cup chicken stock

1 tablespoon parsley, chopped

Directions:

Set the Pressure Pot on Sauté mode, add the oil, heat it, add the fish, and sear for 2 minutes on each side.

Add the rest of the ingredients, put the lid on, and cook on High for 10 minutes.

Release the pressure fast for 5 minutes, divide everything between plates and serve.

Nutrition:

Calories 261, fat 17.6, fiber 2.2, carbs 4.8, protein 22.5.

Steamed Crab Legs

Preparation Time: 12 minutes | Cooking Time: 5 minutes | Servings: 3

Ingredients:

10 oz crab legs

1 cup water, for cooking

Directions:

Pour water and insert the trivet in the Pressure Pot.

Arrange the crab legs on the trivet and close the lid.

Cook the meal on steam mode for 5 minutes.

When the time is over, allow the natural pressure release for 10 minutes.

Remove the cooked crab legs from the Pressure Pot.

Nutrition:

Calories 95, fat 1.4g, fiber 0g, carbs 0g, protein 18.1g.

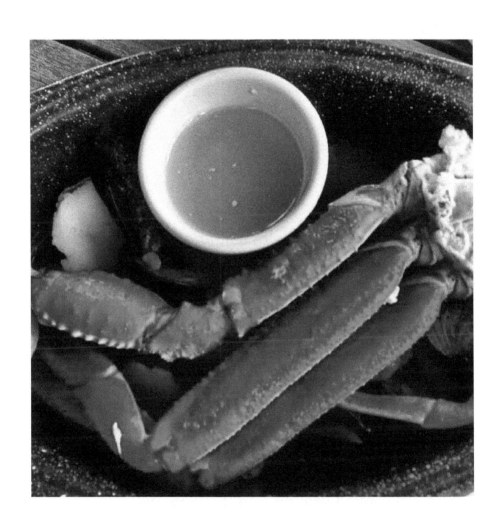

Salmon with Lemon

Preparation Time: 15 minutes | Cooking Time: 10 minutes | Servings: 2

Ingredients:

10 oz salmon fillet

4 lemon slices

1 teaspoon salt

1 teaspoon butter, softened

1 cup water, for cooking

Directions:

Rub the salmon fillet with salt and softened butter.

Then pour water and insert the trivet in the Pressure Pot.

Line the trivet with baking paper and place the salmon fillet on it.

Top the salmon with the lemon slices and close the lid.

Cook the meal for 10 minutes on Steam mode.

When the time is over, allow the natural pressure release and open the lid.

Cut the cooked salmon into the servings.

Nutrition:

Calories 208, fat 10.7g, fiber 0.4g, carbs 1.3g, protein 27.7g.

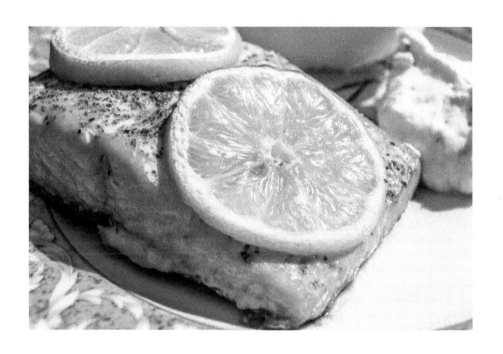

Zingy Fish

Preparation Time: 10 minutes | Cooking Time: 15 minutes | Servings: 4

Ingredients:

1 cup broccoli florets

1-pound coley fillet, chopped

3 tablespoons apple cider vinegar

1 orange slice

1 tablespoon olive oil

1 cup water, for cooking

Directions:

In the mixing bowl combine broccoli florets, coley fillet, apple cider vinegar, and olive oil.

Chop the orange slice and add it to the fish mixture.

Shake the fish mixture well and place it in the Pressure Pot mold.

Pour water and insert the steamer rack.

Place the mold with the fish mixture in the Pressure Pot and close the lid.

Cook the meal on steam mode for 15 minutes.

When the time is over, make a quick pressure release

Nutrition:

Calories 169, fat 4.7g, fiber 0.6g, carbs 4g, protein 26.7g.

Thyme Cod

Preparation Time: 10 minutes | Cooking Time: 10 minutes | Servings: 2

Ingredients:

8 oz cod fillet

1 teaspoon dried thyme

½ teaspoon garlic powder

1 teaspoon sesame oil

1 cup water, for cooking

Directions:

Rub the cod fillet with dried thyme, and garlic powder.

Then sprinkle the fish with sesame oil.

Wrap it in the foil.

Pour water and insert the steamer rack in the Pressure Pot.

Place the wrapped dish in the Pressure Pot and close the lid.

Cook the meal on manual mode (high pressure for 10 minutes.

When the time is over, make a quick pressure release and remove it from the Pressure Pot.

Nutrition:

Calories 115, fat 3.3g, fiber 0.3g, carbs 0.8g, protein 20.4g.

Cajun Salmon with Alfredo Sauce

Preparation Time: 25 minutes | Cooking Time: 10 minutes | Servings: 4

Ingredients:

4 (6-ounce) tilapia fillets, frozen

1 tablespoon of Cajun seasoning

4 tablespoons of unsalted butter

1 cup of heavy cream

½ teaspoon of garlic powder

½ teaspoon of onion powder

½ teaspoon of freshly cracked black pepper

½ teaspoon of fine sea salt

1 cup of parmesan cheese, grated

Directions:

In a heatproof dish that can fit inside your Pressure Pot, add the heavy cream, Cajun seasoning, butter, garlic powder, onion powder, black pepper, salt, and grated parmesan cheese. Stir well.

Place the frozen tilapia fillets on the dish.

Add 2 cups of water and a trivet inside your Pressure Pot.

Place the dish on top of the trivet.

Lock the lid and cook at high pressure for 6 minutes. When the cooking is done, quickly release the pressure and remove the lid. Serve and enjoy!

Nutrition:

Calories 525, Fat 36.2g, Net Carbs 2.9g, Protein 50.4g.

Alaskan Cod with Olives, Fennel, and Cauliflower

Preparation Time: 20 minutes | Cooking Time: 10 minutes | Servings: 3

Ingredients:

2 tablespoons of extra-virgin olive oil

1 pound of Alaskan cod fillet, cut into chunks

½ medium white or yellow onion, chopped

6 garlic cloves, peeled and minced

1 ½ cups of homemade low-sodium chicken stock or fish stock

½ cup of green, black, or Kalamata olives, pitted and chopped

¼ cups of tomato puree

1 head of cauliflower, cut into florets

1 head of fennel, chopped

¼ bunch of fresh basil

1 medium lemon juice

Directions:

Press the "Sauté" setting on your Pressure Pot and add the onions and garlic. Sauté for 5 minutes or until translucent.

Deglaze your Pressure Pot with chicken stock.

Add the remaining ingredients except for the fish and lock the lid. Cook at low pressure for 10 minutes. When the cooking is done, quickly release the pressure and remove the lid.

Press the "Sauté" setting on your Pressure Pot and add the Alaskan cod fillets. Cook for 4 minutes or until the fish is cooked through. Serve and enjoy!

Nutrition:

Calories 201, Fat 15.1g, Net Carbs 6g, Protein 9.3g.

Coconut Fish Curry

Preparation Time: 10 minutes | Cooking Time: 10 minutes | Servings: 4

Ingredients:

1 ½ pound of white fish fillets, cut into bite-sized pieces

1 cup of cherry tomatoes, halved

2 medium red bell peppers, seeds remove and chopped

2 medium onions, thinly sliced

4 garlic cloves, minced

1-inch piece of fresh ginger, peeled and minced

1 teaspoon of fine sea salt

2 tablespoons of olive oil

1 teaspoon of freshly cracked black pepper

2 cups of unsweetened coconut milk

3 tablespoons of madras curry powder

1 lemon, freshly squeezed juice

2 cups of cauliflower rice (for serving)

Directions:

Press the "Sauté" setting on your Pressure Pot and add the olive oil. Once hot, add the onions, ginger, garlic cloves, and red bell pepper. Sauté for 4 to 5 minutes or until translucent.

Add the remaining ingredients and gently stir until well combined.

Lock the lid and cook at high pressure for 3 minutes. When done, quick release the pressure and remove the lid. Serve and enjoy with cauliflower rice!

Nutrition:

Calories 370, Fat 12g, Net Carbs 4g, Protein 43g.

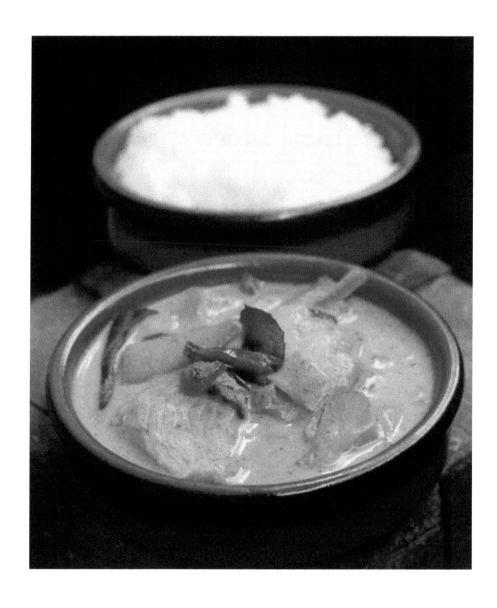

Flavors Parmesan Shrimp

Preparation Time: 10 minutes | Cooking Time: 10 minutes | Servings: 3

Ingredients:

1 lb shrimp, peeled and deveined

1 tbsp olive oil

1/2 tsp onion powder

1/2 tsp basil

1/4 tsp oregano

1/2 tsp pepper

1/4 cup parmesan cheese, grated

3 garlic cloves, minced

Directions:

Add all ingredients into the large bowl and toss well.

Line Pressure Pot multi-level air fryer basket with aluminum foil.

Add shrimp into the air fryer basket and place the basket into the Pressure Pot.

Seal pot with air fryer lid and select air fry mode then set the temperature to 350° F and timer for 10 minutes. Serve and enjoy.

Nutrition:

Calories 251, Fat 8.9g, Carbohydrates 4.2g, Sugar 0.2g, Protein 37.1g, Cholesterol 324mg.

Crispy Coconut Shrimp

Preparation Time: 10 minutes | Cooking Time: 5 minutes | Servings: 2

Ingredients:

8 oz shrimp, peeled

1/4 cup almond flour

2 egg whites

1/8 tsp cayenne pepper

1/4 cup shredded coconut

1/4 tsp salt

Directions:

Whisk egg whites in a shallow dish.

In a bowl, mix the shredded coconut, almond flour, and cayenne pepper.

Place the dehydrating tray in a multi-level air fryer basket and place basket in the Pressure Pot.

Dip shrimp into the egg mixture then coat with coconut mixture and place on dehydrating tray.

Seal pot with air fryer lid and select air fry mode then set the temperature to 400° F and timer for 5 minutes.

Serve and enjoy.

Nutrition:

Calories 272, Fat 12g, Carbohydrates 6.5g, Sugar 0.9g, Protein 32.8g, Cholesterol 239mg.

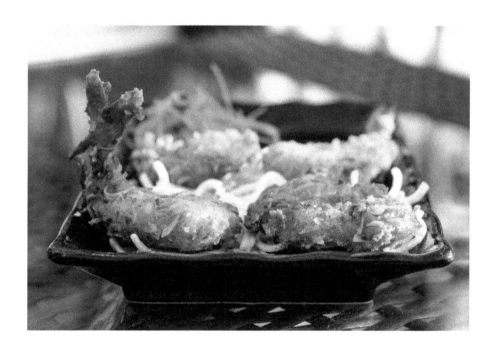

Bacon Wrap Shrimp

Preparation Time: 10 minutes | Cooking Time: 7 minutes | Servings: 2

Ingredients:

8 shrimp, deveined

8 bacon slices

Directions:

Place the dehydrating tray in a multi-level air fryer basket and place basket in the Pressure Pot.

Wrap shrimp with bacon slices and place on dehydrating tray.

Seal pot with air fryer lid and select air fry mode then set the temperature to 390° F and timer for 7 minutes. Turn shrimp after 5 minutes.

Serve and enjoy.

Nutrition:

Calories 516, Fat 33.2g, Carbohydrates 2.4g, Sugar 0g, Protein 48.2g, Cholesterol 269mg.

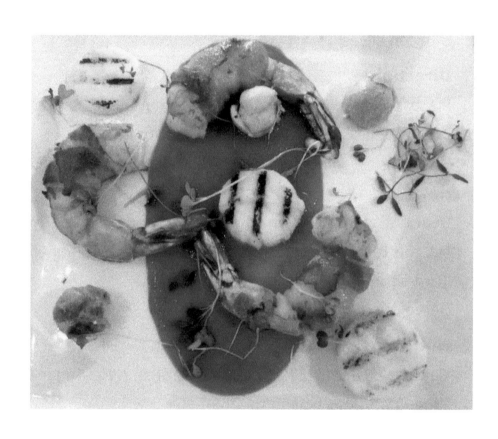

Simple Garlic Lime Shrimp

Preparation Time: 10 minutes | Cooking Time: 8 minutes | Servings: 2

Ingredients:

1 cup shrimp

1 garlic clove, minced

1 fresh lime juice

Pepper

Salt

Directions:

Add all ingredients into the bowl and toss well.

Spray Pressure Pot multi-level air fryer basket with cooking spray.

Add shrimp into the air fryer basket and place the basket into the Pressure Pot.

Seal pot with air fryer lid and select air fry mode then set the temperature to 350° F and timer for 8 minutes.

Turn shrimp halfway through.

Serve and enjoy.

Nutrition:

Calories 201, Fat 2.8g, Carbohydrates 4.9g, Sugar 0.4g, Protein 37.2g, Cholesterol 342mg.

Healthy Catfish

Preparation Time: 10 minutes | Cooking Time: 20 minutes | Servings: 3

Ingredients:

3 catfish fillets

1/4 cup fish seasoning

1 tbsp fresh parsley, chopped

1 tbsp olive oil

Directions:

Place the dehydrating tray in a multi-level air fryer basket and place basket in the Pressure Pot.

Seasoned fish with seasoning and place on dehydrating tray. Brush with olive oil.

Seal pot with air fryer lid and select air fry mode then set the temperature to 400° F and timer for 20 minutes.

Turn fish fillets halfway through.

Garnish with parsley and serve.

Nutrition:

Calories 286, Fat 16.8g, Carbohydrates 6.1g, Sugar 0g, Protein 24.9g, Cholesterol 75mg.

Lemon Crab Patties

Preparation Time: 10 minutes | Cooking Time: 10 minutes | Servings: 4

Ingredients:

1 egg

12 oz crabmeat

2 green onion, chopped

1/4 cup mayonnaise

1 cup almond flour

1 tsp old bay seasoning

1 tsp red pepper flakes

1 tbsp fresh lemon juice

Directions:

Add half almond flour into the shallow bowl.

Add remaining ingredients and mix until well combined.

Place the dehydrating tray in a multi-level air fryer basket and place basket in the Pressure Pot.

Make patties and coat with remaining almond flour and place on dehydrating tray.

Seal pot with air fryer lid and select air fry mode then set the temperature to 400° F and timer for 10 minutes.

Turn patties halfway through.

Serve and enjoy.

Nutrition:

Calories 327, Fat 19.8g, Carbs 23.2g, Sugar 6.6g, Protein 14.2g, Cholesterol 62mg.

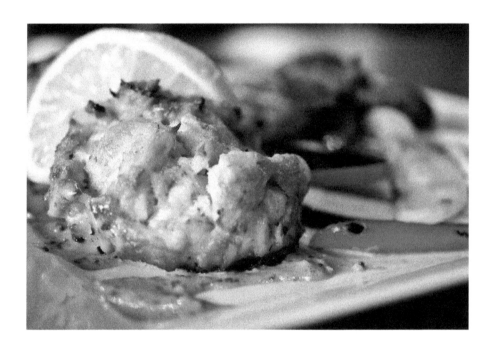

Cheese Crust Salmon

Preparation Time: 10 minutes | Cooking Time: 10 minutes | Servings: 2

Ingredients:

2 salmon fillets

2 tbsp fresh parsley, chopped

1 garlic clove, minced

1/4 cup parmesan cheese, shredded

1/2 tsp McCormick's BBQ seasoning

1/2 tsp paprika

1 tbsp olive oil

Pepper

Salt

Directions:

Add salmon, seasoning, and olive oil to the bowl and mix well.

Mix cheese, garlic, and parsley.

Sprinkle cheese mixture on top of salmon.

Place the dehydrating tray in a multi-level air fryer basket and place basket in the Pressure Pot.

Place salmon fillets on a dehydrating tray.

Seal pot with air fryer lid and select air fry mode then set the temperature to 400° F and timer for 10 minutes.

Serve and enjoy.

Nutrition:

Calories 341, Fat 20.5g, Carbohydrates 2.2g, Sugar 0.6g, Protein 38.5g, Cholesterol 87mg.

Shredded pork

Preparation time: 10 minutes | Cooking Time: 30 minutes | Servings: 4

Ingredients:

2 lbs. pork shoulder

1/2 tsp oregano

1 onion, chopped

2 lime juice

1/2 cup of water

2 cups chicken broth

1 tbsp olive oil

2 garlic cloves, minced

1/2 tsp cumin

Directions:

Add oil into the Pressure Pot and set the pot on sauté mode.

Add meat to the pot and sauté until browned.

Add remaining ingredients to the pot and stir well.

Seal pot with lid and cook on manual high pressure for 30 minutes.

Once done then allow to release pressure naturally then open the lid.

Shred the meat using a fork and serve.

Nutrition:

Calories 732, Fat 52.8g, Carbohydrates 5.6g, Sugar 1.9g, Protein 55.8g, Cholesterol 204mg.

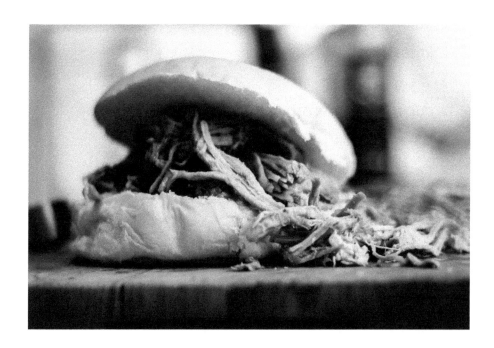

Pork Curry

Preparation time: 10 minutes | Cooking Time: 37 minutes | Servings: 8

Ingredients:

4 lbs. pork shoulder, boneless and cut into chunks

2 garlic cloves, minced

1 onion, chopped

3 cups chicken broth

2 cups of coconut milk

1/2 tsp turmeric

2 tbsp olive oil

1/2 tbsp ground cumin

1 1/2 tbsp curry paste

2 tbsp fresh ginger, grated

Pepper

Salt

Directions:

Add oil into the pot and set the pot on sauté mode.

Season meat with pepper and salt. Add meat to the pot and cook until browned.

Add remaining ingredients and stir everything well.

Seal pot with lid and cook on soup/stew mode for 30 minutes.

Once done then release pressure using the quick-release method then open the lid.

Stir well and serve.

Nutrition:

Calories 877, Fat 68.6g, Carbohydrates 7.2g, Sugar 2.9g, Protein 56.5g, Cholesterol 204mg.

Meatloaf

Preparation time: 10 minutes | Cooking Time: 45 minutes | Servings: 6

Ingredients:

2 1/4 lbs ground beef

1 tsp thyme

1 1/2 cups water

2 eggs, lightly beaten

3 tbsp olive oil

1/2 tsp garlic salt

1 tsp rosemary

1/4 tsp sage

1 tsp parsley

1 tsp oregano

Directions:

Pour water into the Pressure Pot and place trivet in the pot.

Spray loaf pan with cooking spray.

Add all ingredients into the bowl and mix until combined.

Pour the meat mixture into the loaf pan and place the pan on top of the trivet.

Seal pot with lid and cook on manual high pressure for 30 minutes.

Once done then allow to release pressure naturally for 10 minutes then release using the quick-release method. Open the lid.

Serve and enjoy.

Nutrition:

Calories 400, Fat 19.1g, Carbohydrates 0.7g, Sugar 0.2g, Protein 53.6g, Cholesterol 207mg.

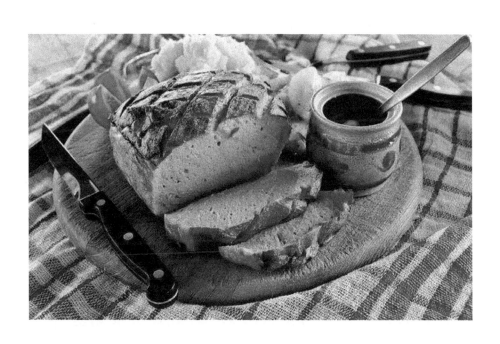

Cajun Beef

Preparation time: 10 minutes | Cooking Time: 12 minutes | Servings: 4

Ingredients:

1 lb ground beef

1 cup beef broth

10 oz Mexican cheese

1 tbsp olive oil

2 tbsp tomato paste

1 1/2 tbsp cajun seasoning

Directions:

Add oil into the Pressure Pot and set the pot on sauté mode.

Add meat to the pot and sauté until browned.

Add cajun seasoning, broth, and tomato paste. Stir well.

Seal pot with lid and cook on manual high pressure for 7 minutes.

Release pressure using the quick-release method than open the lid.

Add cheese and stir well. Cover the pot again and cook on manual high pressure for 5 minutes.

Once done then release pressure using the quick-release method then open the lid.

Stir and serve.

Nutrition:

Calories 510, Fat 33.7g, Carbs 4.3g, Sugar 1.1g, Protein 51.2g, Cholesterol 165mg.

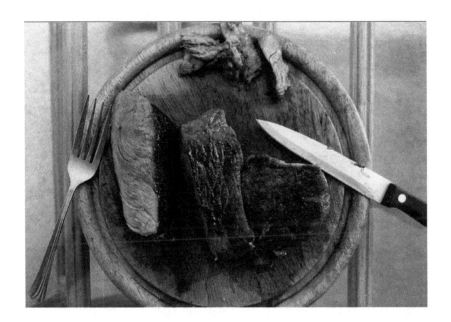

Cheesy Beef

Preparation time: 10 minutes | Cooking Time: 22 minutes | Servings: 4

Ingredients:

1 lb ground beef

13.5 oz can tomato, diced

1/2 cup mozzarella cheese, shredded

1/2 cup tomato puree

1 tsp basil

1 tsp oregano

1 tbsp olive oil

1/2 onion, diced

1 carrot, sliced

Directions:

Add oil into the Pressure Pot and set the pot on sauté mode.

Add onion to the pot and sauté for 2-3 minutes.

Add meat and cook until browned.

Add tomatoes, oregano, basil, and tomato puree. Stir well.

Seal pot with lid and cook on manual high pressure for 15 minutes.

Once done then release pressure using the quick-release method then open the lid.

Set pot on sauté mode. Add cheese and cook for 5 minutes.

Serve and enjoy.

Nutrition:

Calories 296, Fat 11.3g, Carbohydrates 10.9g, Sugar 6.1g, Protein 37.1g, Cholesterol 103mg.

Coriander Cod Mix

Preparation time: 5 minutes | Cooking Time: 15 minutes | Servings: 4

Ingredients:

4 cod fillets, boneless and skinless

1 cup coconut cream

2 spring onions, sliced

2 garlic cloves, minced

1 tablespoons coriander, chopped

A pinch of salt and black pepper

2 tablespoons lime juice

Directions:

In your Pressure Pot, combine the trout with the cream and the rest of the ingredients, put the lid on and cook on High for 15 minutes.

Release the pressure fast for 5 minutes, divide everything between plates and serve.

Nutrition:

Calories 297, fat 24.3g, fiber 1.6g, carbs 5.4g, protein 17.6g.

Cod and Zucchinis

Preparation time: 5 minutes | Cooking Time: 15 minutes | Servings: 4

Ingredients:

4 cod fillets, boneless and skinless

2 zucchinis, sliced

1 tablespoon avocado oil

2 garlic cloves, minced

1 tablespoon sweet paprika

Salt and black pepper to the taste

1 tablespoon parsley, chopped

½ cup veggie stock

Directions:

Set the Pressure Pot on Sauté mode, add the oil, heat it, add the garlic and sauté for 2 minutes.

Add the rest of the ingredients, put the lid on, and cook on High for 12 minutes.

Release the pressure naturally for 5 minutes, divide the mix between plates and serve.

Nutrition:

Calories 182, fat 10.4g, fiber 1.9g, carbs 6.2g, protein 17.5g.

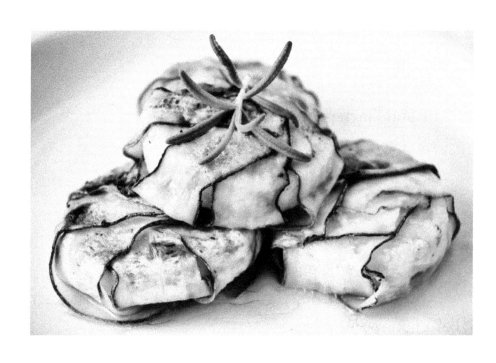

Paprika Trout

Preparation time: 5 minutes | Cooking Time: 12 minutes | Servings: 4

Ingredients:

4 trout fillets, boneless and skinless

½ cup chicken stock

A pinch of salt and black pepper

½ teaspoon oregano, dried

2 teaspoons sweet paprika

1 tablespoon chives, chopped

Directions:

In your Pressure Pot, combine the trout with the rest of the ingredients, put the lid on, and cook on High for 12 minutes.

Release the pressure fast for 5 minutes, divide the mix between plates and serve.

Nutrition:

Calories 132, fat 5.5g, fiber 0.5g, carbs 0.9g, protein 16.8g.

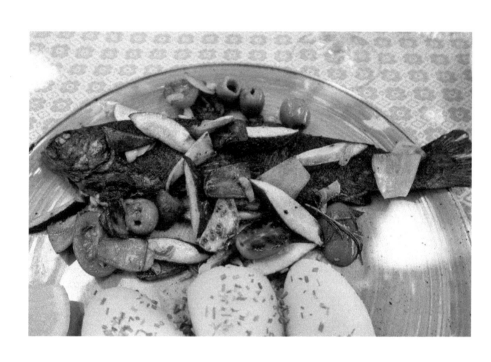

Lime Shrimp

Preparation time: 5minutes | Cooking Time: 8 minutes | Servings: 4

Ingredients:

1 pound shrimp, peeled and deveined

Zest of 1 lime, grated

Juice of 1 lime

1 cup chicken stock

¼ cup cilantro, chopped

A pinch of salt and black pepper

Directions:

In your Pressure Pot, combine the shrimp with the rest of the ingredients, put the lid on, and cook on High for 8 minutes.

Release the pressure fast for 5 minutes, divide the shrimp between plates and serve with a side salad.

Nutrition:

Calories 138, fat 3.8g, fiber 0g, carbs 2g, protein 26g.

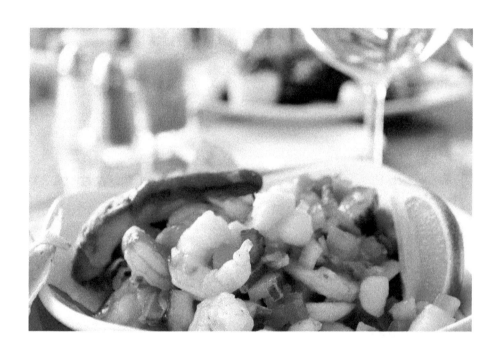

Pork Patties

Preparation Time: 10 minutes | Cooking Time: 15 minutes | Servings: 6

Ingredients:

2 lbs ground pork

1 tsp red pepper flakes

1 tbsp dried parsley

1 1/2 tbsp Italian seasoning

1 tsp fennel seed

1 tsp paprika

2 tbsp olive oil

2 tsp salt

Directions:

Line Pressure Pot air fryer basket with parchment paper.

In a large bowl, mix ground pork, fennel seed, paprika, red pepper flakes, parsley, Italian seasoning, olive oil, pepper, and salt.

Make small patties from the meat mixture and place them on parchment paper into the air fryer basket.

Place basket into the pot.

Seal the pot with an air fryer basket and select bake mode and cook at 375° F for 15 minutes.

Serve and enjoy.

Nutrition:

Calories 270, Fat 11.2g, Carbohydrates 1g, Sugar 0.4g, Protein 39.7g, Cholesterol 113mg.

Herb Pork Tenderloin

Preparation Time: 10 minutes | Cooking Time: 30 minutes | Servings: 4

Ingredients:

1 lb pork tenderloin

1 tsp oregano, dried

1 tsp thyme, dried

1 tsp olive oil

1/2 tsp onion powder

1/2 tsp garlic powder

1/2 tsp pepper

1/2 tsp salt

Directions:

In a small bowl, mix onion powder, garlic powder, oregano, thyme, pepper, and salt.

Coat pork with oil then rubs with herb mixture and place into the Pressure Pot air fryer basket.

Place basket in the pot.

Seal the pot with an air fryer lid and select roast mode and cook at 400 ° F for 30 minutes.

Slice and serve.

Nutrition:

Calories 177, Fat 5.2g, Carbohydrates 1.1g, Sugar 0.2g, Protein 29.9g, Cholesterol 83mg.

Buttery Pork Chops

Preparation Time: 10 minutes | Cooking Time: 10 minutes | Servings: 6

Ingredients:

6 pork chops, boneless

1 stick butter

1 tbsp olive oil

1 cup of water

1 tbsp ranch seasoning

Directions

Add oil into the inner pot of Pressure Pot duo crisp and set pot on sauté mode.

Add pork chops and cook until brown. Sprinkle ranch seasoning over pork chops then add butter.

Pour water over pork chops.

Seal the pot with a pressure-cooking lid and cook on high for 5 minutes.

Once done, allow to release pressure naturally. Remove lid.

Serve and enjoy.

Nutrition:

Calories 410, Fat 37g, Carbohydrates 2g, Sugar 1g, Protein 18g, Cholesterol 105mg.

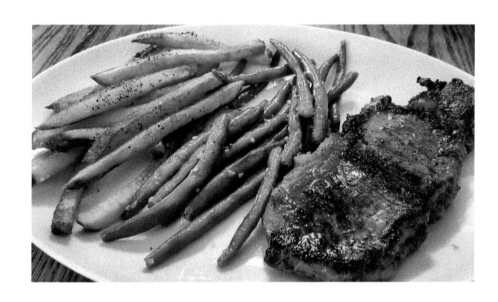

Tasty Boneless Pork Chops

Preparation Time: 10 minutes | Cooking Time: 15 minutes | Servings: 2

Ingredients:

2 pork chops, boneless

1/4 cup beef broth

2 tbsp lemon pepper

¼ tsp garlic powder

Directions:

Set Pressure Pot duo crisp on sauté mode.

Place pork chops into the inner pot of Pressure Pot and season with garlic powder and lemon pepper.

Cook pork chops until brown.

Remove pork chops from the pot. Add broth and deglaze the pan.

Return pork chops into the pot.

Seal the pot with a pressure-cooking lid and cook on high for 10 minutes.

Once done, allow to release pressure naturally. Remove lid.

Serve and enjoy.

Nutrition:

Calories 285, Fat 20g, Carbohydrates 7g, Protein 18.7g, Sugar 3g, Cholesterol 69mg.

Chipotle Beef

Preparation Time: 10 minutes | Cooking Time: 1 hour 40 minutes | Servings: 4

Ingredients:

3 1/2 lbs beef brisket, cut into pieces

2 tbsp chipotle powder

¼ tsp garlic powder

1 tbsp butter

1/4 cup cilantro, chopped

1 cup chicken broth

1 tsp sea salt

Directions:

Add butter into the inner pot of Pressure Pot duo crisp and set pot on sauté mode.

Add meat and sauté until lightly brown.

Add remaining ingredients and stir well.

Seal the pot with a pressure-cooking lid and cook on high for 1 hour 40 minutes.

Once done, release pressure using a quick release. Remove lid.

Slice and serve.

Nutrition:

Calories 764, Fat 26g, Carbohydrates 0.2g, Protein 121g, Sugar 0.2g, Cholesterol 360mg.

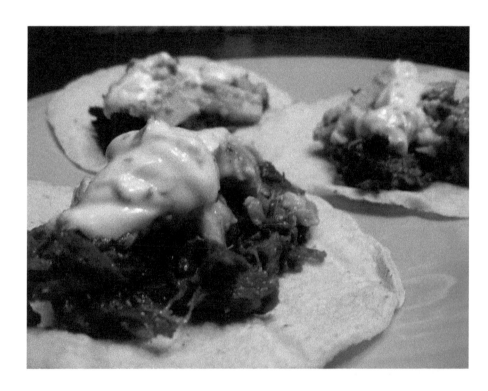

Delicious Picadillo

Preparation Time: 10 minutes | Cooking Time: 15 minutes | Servings: 6

Ingredients:

2 lbs ground beef

14 oz can roast tomatoes, blended

2 cups cherry tomatoes, halved

1 bell pepper, diced

1/2 cup green olives

1/2 tsp ground cumin

1/2 cup green onion, chopped

1 tbsp olive oil

1 tsp salt

Directions:

Add oil into the inner pot of Pressure Pot duo crisp and set pot on sauté mode.

Add meat and cook until browned, about 5 minutes.

Add remaining ingredients and stir well.

Seal the pot with a pressure-cooking lid and cook on high for 10 minutes.

Once done, release pressure using a quick release. Remove lid.

Stir well and serve.

Nutrition:

Calories 348, Fat 13g, Carbs 8g, Sugar 5g, Protein 47g, Cholesterol 135mg.

Lamb Patties

Preparation Time: 10 minutes | Cooking Time: 12 minutes | Servings: 6

Ingredients:

1 lb ground lamb

1 tsp dried rosemary

1 tbsp dried oregano

1 tbsp dried thyme

1 lb ground beef

1/4 cup green onion, chopped

2 tbsp olive oil

1 tsp cumin

1 tsp pepper

1 1/2 tsp salt

Directions:

Add all ingredients into the large bowl and mix until combined.

Make small patties from the meat mixture.

Place patties in an Pressure Pot air fryer basket and place basket in the pot.

Seal the pot with an air fryer lid and select bake mode and cook at 360° F for 12 minutes.

Serve and enjoy.

Nutrition:

Calories 329, Fat 15g, Carbs 1.6g, Sugar 0.2g, Protein 44g, Cholesterol 136mg.

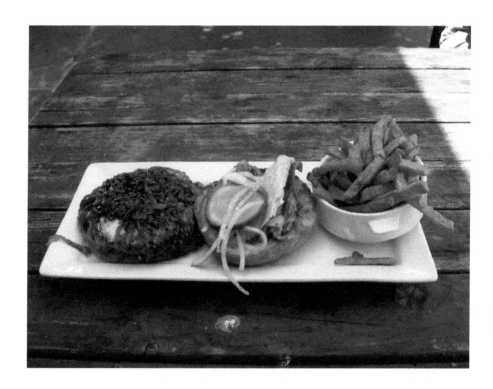

Ranch Seasoned Pork Chops

Preparation Time: 10 minutes | Cooking Time: 35 minutes | Servings: 6

Ingredients:

6 pork chops, boneless

1/4 cup olive oil

1 tsp dried parsley

2 tbsp ranch seasoning, homemade

Pepper

Salt

Directions:

Season pork chops with pepper and salt and place into the Pressure Pot air fryer basket. Place basket in the pot.

Mix olive oil, parsley, and ranch seasoning.

Brush pork chops with oil mixture.

Seal the pot with an air fryer lid and select bake mode and cook at 400° F for 30-35 minutes.

Serve and enjoy.

Nutrition:

Calories 328, Fat 28g, Carbohydrates 0g, Sugar 0g, Protein 18g, Cholesterol 69mg.

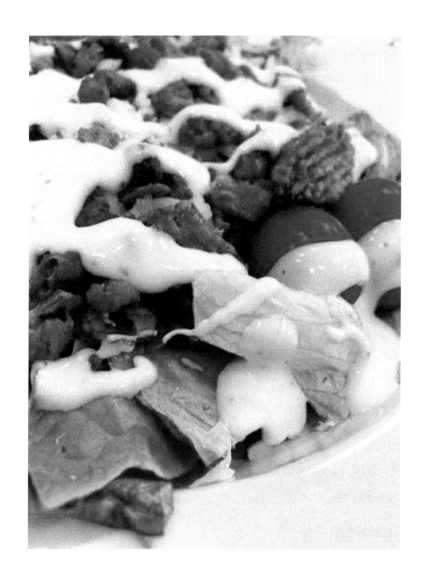

Lightning Source UK Ltd.
Milton Keynes UK
UKHW020808180621
385732UK00001B/75